Repellents:

DIY Non-Toxic Repellent Recipes To Protect Your Family And Yourself From Mosquitos And Ants

Table of Contents:

Repellents: 1

DIY Non-Toxic Repellent Recipes To Protect Your Family And Yourself From Mosquitos And Ants 1

Introduction 3

Chapter 1 – Essential Tools for Natural Insect Repellents 5

Chapter 2 – Non-Toxic Repellents for Ants...11

Chapter 3 – Natural Repellents for Mosquito...17

Chapter 4 – Get Rid of Roaches and Dust Mites 22

Chapter 5 – Natural and Non-Toxic Repellent for Kids and Pets.............26

Conclusion 33

Introduction

With the increasing threat of West Nile disease and Lyme virus, many people feel that it is essential to use insect repellents. The use of insect repellents is particularly important in the areas where these viruses and illnesses prevail.

Commercial repellents can be harmful to you and your family because these often contain chemicals and fragrances. Its components and substance can irritate your sensitive skin and have an unpleasant odor. You can get the advantage of insect homemade insect repellents. These repellents are made of natural ingredients that are non-toxic and safe. These are free from unpleasant odor and dangerous ingredients.

There are lots of options to make homemade repellent and you can test the effectiveness of these repellents. Homemade bug repellent is good to use in the outside events, garden work, picnic and patio. Chemical based insect repellents can be too strong with harmful substances.

There is no need to use chemical bug repellents because you can make your own natural repellent to get rid of bugs and insects. The homemade spray is the best alternative of commercial repellents. You can make a blend of different types of oils, lotions, and other items. Homemade insect sprays are free from toxins and you can use them without any danger.

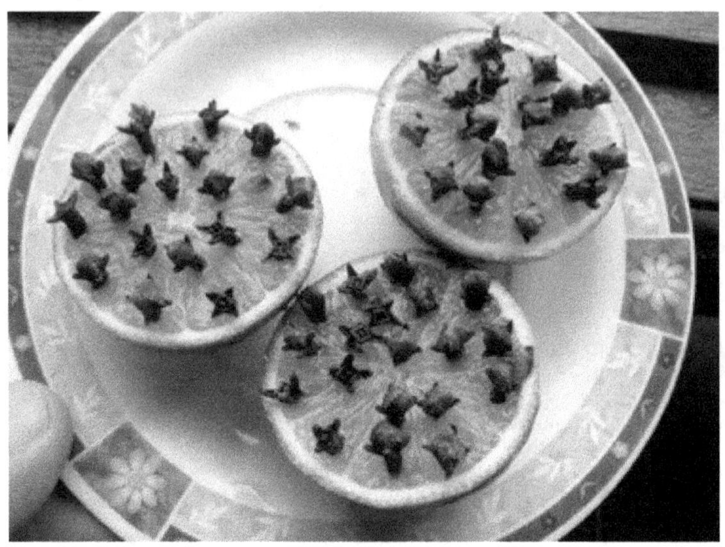

With the help of essential oils, you can make a spray with the pleasant smell to keep the insects at bay. These sprays will provide a pleasant smell to your home and always keep you calm.

There are numerous herbs and essential oils that can be used to get the advantage of its amazing smell. There are numerous ways to get the advantage of plants around your house. It is essential to use these natural ingredients to design these sprays. This book is designed for your assistance with a lot of natural and non-toxic ant and mosquito repellents. These recipes are simple to follow and easy to make.

Read this book and learn different ways to prepare insect repellents. Make sure to follow these recipes and get rid of chemical-based insect repellents.

Chapter 1 – Essential Tools for Natural Insect Repellents

Before making natural insect repellents, you should get all important materials ready. You may need two tablespoons of witch hazel, vodka or both. It is essential to use two tablespoons of any neem oil, jojoba oil, olive oil, grapeseed oil and various other essential oils with natural insecticidal qualities.

You can prepare half teaspoon vodka, 110 drops of high-quality essential oils. Almost 55 drops of eucalyptus lemon oil are an excellent alternative to DEET that is used to repel insects and bugs. You can also use 15 drops pure lavender oil and 15 drops cedar wood oil. Rosemary essential oil is another choice to get rid of insects naturally.

You can dilute essential oils with carrier oils and pour these oils in a small spray bottle with the 1/4th capacity to shake this liquid. It is easy to apply essential oils on your skin for a few hours for the best results.

Homemade Repellent Lotions for Kids

These lotions are friendly and work effectively against insects and bugs. These are good to keep your skin healthy, such as coconut oil feeds vitamin E to your skin. Pure coconut oil is available in the market and you can apply it on your skin. Take a 1/3rd cup of coconut oil, 15 drops clove oil, peppermint oil or lavender oil to make a homemade repellent. Mix these ingredients, shake well and apply on the skin of your children. You can use a big spray bottle to spray this solution in your room.

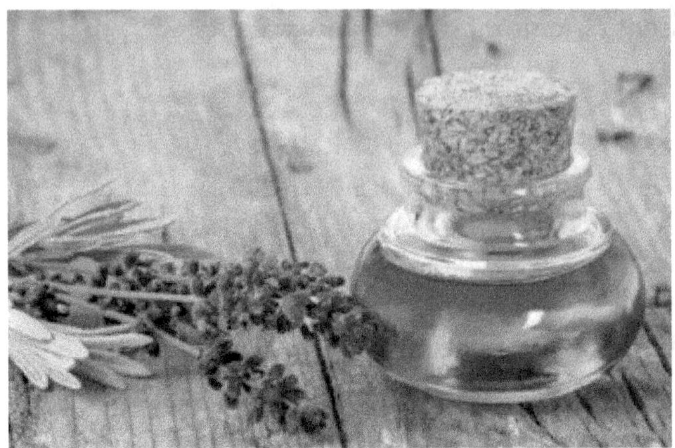

You can rub this solution on the legs, arms and exposed body parts of your children. There is no problem, if this lotion gets in the mouth of your children because it is non-toxic, but you should remove it immediately.

Repellent Lotions for Adults

If you want strong lotion, you can prepare a lotion with 1/3rd cup of castile soap in liquid form. It is available in eucalyptus, tea tree, and citrus oils. You can take 30 drops of oils of your preference and mix it with liquid castile soap. Shake well in a bottle to apply on your legs, neck, hairline and among other parts of the body.

Apply this lotion on your skin before going toward the woods, in a campsite and garden. Keep it in mind to apply it on your skin after every few hours to protect it against all insects. After heading back to home, you should wash the lotion properly. It is effective to keep all bugs away and good to soap the user up at the time of the bath.

Repellent Spray for Kids and Pets

Pets and children have sensitive skin and you should be careful while making insect spray. You can prepare spray for small kids with witch hazel, lemongrass, clove, lavender or peppermint essential oil. For older pets and kids, you can use tea tree oil, eucalyptus and lemon. Keep it in mind that lemon and eucalyptus oil is not good for small children. It can cause irritation on their skin.

You can start with hazel and water mixture and add 15 drops oil in the mixture. Shake this lotion well before use and spray to get best results in every three to four hours. This spray can be used on arms, legs, back and neck of small children.

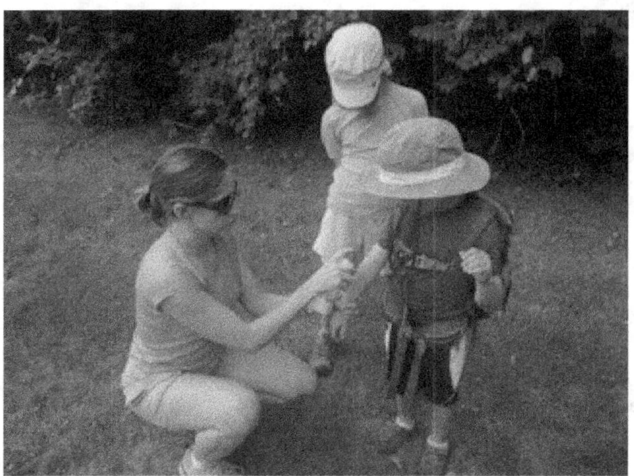

To protect your children from insects and bugs, keep them away from forested areas and stagnant water. If they like to play in the garden, you can treat the selected area with the smoke of cedar wood. You should set up traps for bugs around your children and pay attention to the skin of your children.

For pets, the spray can be used on legs, around collar and tails. You can use pure citronella, tea tree and eucalyptus oils on the collar to keep biters away from your pets.

Adults Sprays

If you want to make a stronger version of spray for adults, you can use water, lemon oil, hazel, tea tree oil, citronella oil and eucalyptus oil. Vegetable glycerine is also useful to make this spray. Start your work with the combination of 20:80 water and witch hazel.

Make sure to add one teaspoon vegetable glycerine and 30 drops of your favorite essential oil. Use this spray before hiking and mountain climbing. This natural spray will protect you from annoying bugs and insects. For a better protection, you can prepare a combination of tea tree, lemon, and eucalyptus. It may have a negative reaction on your skin; therefore, test it on your skin before using it.

Possible Side Effects of Herbal Remedies

Some medicinal herbs are very good for your health because these are highly recommended for the various mental and other health conditions. There are some rare side effects that are associated with their use:

Allergic Reactions

Just like any modern drugs, the herbal medicines also have adverse effects on the body, such as these can cause allergic reactions. Sometimes the combination of some herbs can be the reason of allergic reactions. It is really important to be careful about different combinations because some combinations can be toxic for your health.

Herbal Drugs have Not been Regulated

Unlike any other traditional medicinal drug, the natural drugs are not regulated by the Food and Drug Authority. They are often considered as dietary supplements. Due to their dietary supplement status, it is considered that these are allowed to sell safely anywhere. These are safe and effective, but be careful while purchasing and make sure to consult a naturopath for your help.

It can Interact with Drugs

The herbs can also interact with the traditional drug because of its natural properties. It can amplify the effects of medication, or can reduce its effects to make it dangerous. You need to tell your doctor that you are using, these herbs before following any prescription.

It can be the reason of Unwanted Conditions

There are few medicinal herbs that can make your health conditions worse. The Tarragon should be used with extreme care because it is not good for the people suffering from any kind of cancer. The mistletoe is not good for the use of pregnant women because it can lead her to miscarriage.

The natural herbs are good to treat various ailments, and these are low in cost too. You can buy them from any herbal medicinal drug store, food shop, and any other pharmacies. These may have some unwanted health effects while combining with traditional drugs. You can consult a naturopath and a herbalist to get a right combination. You need to tell your doctor that you are going to take an alternative.

Chapter 2 – Non-Toxic Repellents for Ants

Ants live in colonies to work together, forage for food and water to survive in a cold environment. Ants can be a real irritation in your house because you can find them in the kitchen, bedroom, living room, etc. They can destroy your plants and food items in your house. People often use a chemical at repellents, but these are toxic and harmful to your pets and children. You can prepare homemade repellents and spray them directly in your house. There are a few recipes given for your assistance:

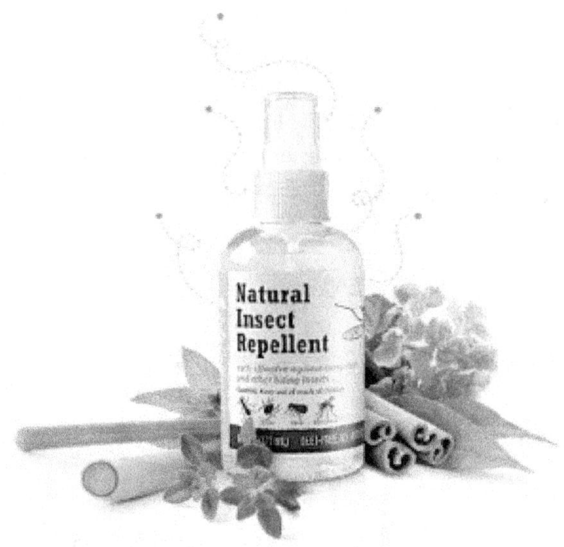

Recipe 01: Insect Repellent

- Water and vinegar 50/50 mixture

- Lavender or tea tree oil: 30 drops

- Witch hazel: 1 tablespoon

You a prepare a mixture of all these ingredients and prepare your own ant repellent spray.

Recipe 02: Jam Bait

- TBC Borax or Boric Acid

- Jelly, maple syrup or honey

Directions:

Prepare a mixture of jam and boric acid to prepare a paste. Now, slather this paste on a piece of paper or a container having holes. You can increase the amount of boric acid to make this paste strong.

Recipe 03: Sugar Baits

- Sugar: 2 cups

- Water: 1 cup

- Boric Acid: 2 tablespoons

Directions:

Prepare this mixture and prepare it in a small saucer all the way around your house.

Recipe 04: Protein Baits

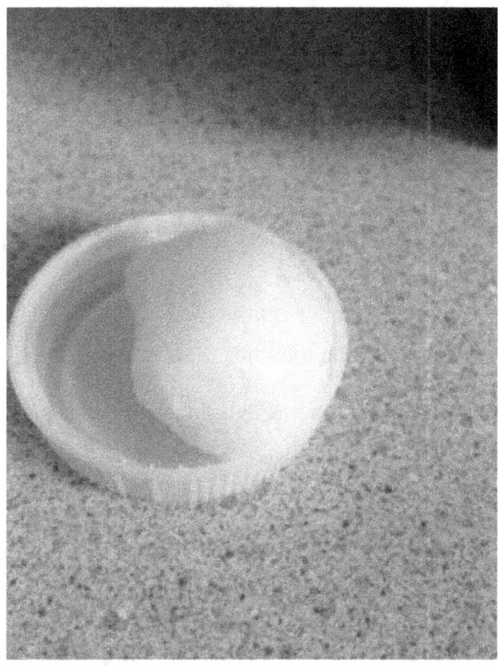

- Bacon grease or peanut butter

- 2 tablespoons boric acid

Directions:

Prepare this mixture and mount it on a piece of paper.

Recipe 05: Destroy Their Nests

It is essential to find the nests of ants and pour the following solution on the nests. Make sure to wear rubber boots and legs to avoid any problem:

- ¼ cup dish detergent to one gallon boiling water (always add soap after removing it from the stove). This solution is excellent for fire ants

- You can pour cider vinegar inside their nests to kill them, but this can kill your grass and plants too.

- Mix salt in boiling water to make a strong solution and pour it on the nests. Replicate it for three days and avoid rebuilding nests in this area.

- Try to disturb their dwelling on a regular basis and flood the areas with water using a garden hose.

Recipe 06: Orange Peels for Ants

With the help of orange peels, you can repel ants and kill them. For this work, you will need:

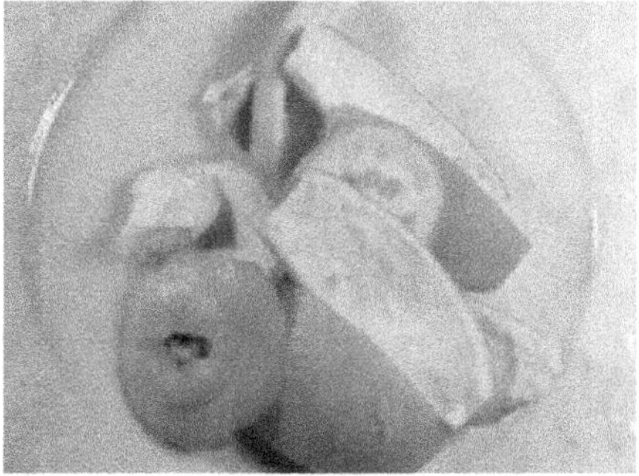

- Blender

- Water

- Orange peels

Directions:

Pour one cup water and orange peels in a blender and make a blend. You can increase the amount of this blend and pour this solution on the hills of ants to kill them.

To make your work easy, dump this solution in any spray container and use it to spray any affected area in your home to kill ants. It will be good to spray this solution in the outer base of your house to block the ways of ants from entering your house.

Recipe 07: Natural Ant Repellent

- Black Pepper powder

- Cinnamon

- Bay Leaves

- Ground red Chili

- Cucumber Peels

- Whole Cloves

- Red Pepper Flakes

- Coffee Grounds

- Salt

- Sage

- Various Essential Oils: Lavender, Peppermint, and Eucalyptus. You can swab these oils on entrance points.

Tip: You can fill Vaseline in the cracks and holes to block physical entry of ants.

Chapter 3 – Natural Repellents for Mosquito

Insect repellent is a substance to apply on your cloth or skin to discourage insects and control them. There are some special essential oils that will help you to make mosquito repellent sprays:

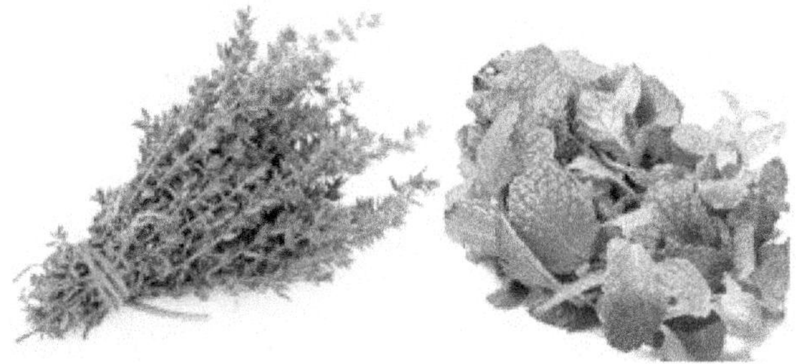

Recipe 07: Natural Inset Repellent Spray

- 2 ounces boiled or distilled water

- Citronella oil: 30 drops

- Vodka or witch hazel: 1.5 ounces

- Peppermint oil: 25 drops

- Tea tree oil: 15 drops

Jojoba oil: 1 teaspoon (If you want to add this, you should add 1-ounce witch hazel or vodka)

Directions:

You will need 4 ounces spray bottle and fill it with water. Now, add vodka or witch hazel along with 50 to 75 drops of essential oils. Shake it well and spray this mixture on the exposed clothing and skin. Avoid its use to eyes and keep this bottle away from sunlight and heat. Apply it once again after every two hours. Make sure to buy therapeutic grade essential oils.

Recipe 08: Essential Oil Blends

- Cedarwood: 10 drops

- Rosemary: 10 drops

- Lavender: 10 drops

- Lemon Eucalyptus: 30 drops

Directions:

Prepare a mixture of these oils, add your favorite witch hazel and use as an insect repellent lotion. Apply it on your skin to get rid of mosquito. This repellent is not safe for the children under 3.

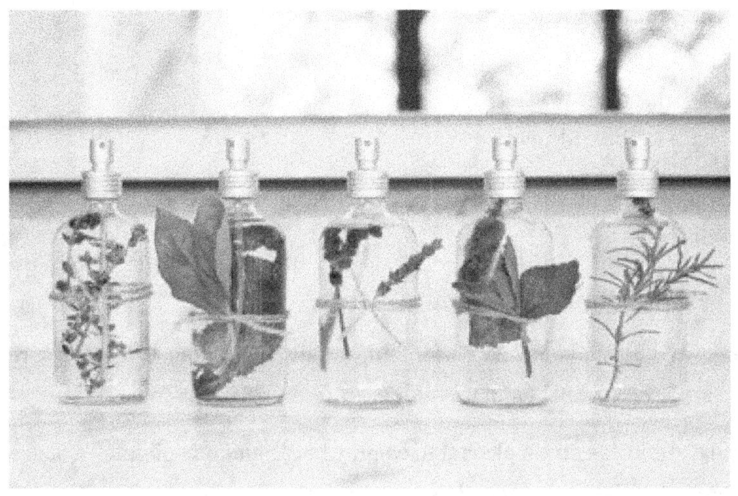

Recipe 09: Lavender Mosquito Repellent

- 3 to 4 tablespoons vanilla extract

- 15 drops lavender oil

- Distilled water

- ¼ cup lemon juice

Directions:

Pour all these ingredients in a spray bottle and shake well to combine this mixture. You can spray it on skin and clothes. This spray remains good for almost six months.

Recipe 10: Cloves Repellent

- 3.5-ounce cloves

- 16-ounce rubbing alcohol

- 3.5-ounce baby oil (or you can use lavender, chamomile, sesame, almond or fennel oils)

Directions:

Put cloves in your alcohol and leave it for almost four days to infuse it. Make sure to stir cloves on every evening and morning.

After four days, you can strain alcohol in a spray bottle and mix oil into it. Shake it well before use and spray this on clothing and skin.

Recipe 11: Tick and Mosquito Repellent

- 2-ounce castor oil

- 6-ounce witch hazel

- Eucalyptus oil: 15 drops

- Cinnamon oil: 5 drops

- Citronella oil: 15 drops

Directions:

Pour all these ingredients in a spray bottle and shake well to combine this mixture. You can spray it on skin and clothes. This spray remains good for almost six months.

Recipe 12: Stop Pain and Itch of Mosquito Bite

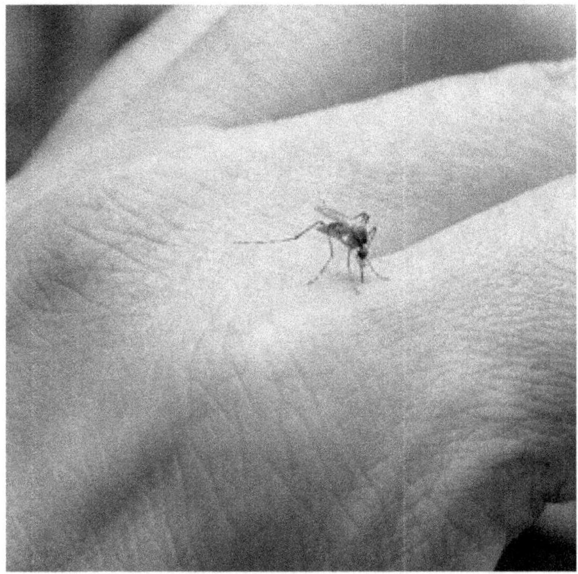

- You can apply tea tree or lavender oil to the insect bite.

- Apple cider vinegar is also good to apply to the mosquito bite.

- Lemon slice can be rubbed on the affected area.

- You can apply ice cubes on the mosquito bite.

- Tea bags of chamomile will help you to diminish inflammation and soothe the pain.

- A paste of baking soda and water can be applied to the affected skin.

- One slice of onion can immediately reduce pain and inflammation of insect bites.

Chapter 4 – Get Rid of Roaches and Dust Mites

Roaches and dust mites are really harmful to your health because these can pollute the environment of your house. There are a few recipes to get rid of roaches:

Recipe 13: Bay Leaves

You can use bay leaves because its fragrance can keep the roaches away. Take a few bay leaves and crush these leaves because essential oils of these leaves will give a strong fragrance. These crushed leaves can be tucked into the cushions of the beds and the corners of the shelf. It will make roaches immediately run away from the place. It will help you to remove roaches from your house.

Recipe 14: Sugar and Baking Soda

Take baking soda and sugar in equal quantities and prepare a mixture. Apply this mixture in an area where you frequently find roaches. Sugar will attract roaches and they may eat it. The baking soda will upset the stomach of roaches and slowly kill them.

Recipe 15: Garlic, Pepper, and Onion Solution

You can take one-liter water in a mug and add one tablespoon powder of cayenne pepper, one clove of garlic and paste of one onion. Marinate this mixture for one hour and pour one teaspoon solution of liquid soap in this mixture. Apply this mixture to all places where you see roaches frequently.

Recipe 16: Trap of Petroleum Jelly

Use a jar and apply petroleum jelly to the inside border of the jar. You can put the peels of a few fruits, such as mango, apple, and banana for the strong smell. Keep this solution in the area where you notice roaches because the sweet smell will attract roaches in the jar, but the petroleum jelly will trap them. After trapping roaches, discard the content of the jar in a bucket of soapy water and flush it down the toilet.

Recipe 17: Simple Remedies for Dust Mites

- Use dust mite protective covers and wash your bed sheets and pillows with hot water almost once a week.

- Keep your pillows in the freezer for almost few hours once in a month.

- Evaporates humidity of bed because dust mites love humidity and airing will destroy them.

- Make a dust mite repellent spray with lavender, clove, Eucalyptus, Rosemary and Peppermint. Mix a few drops of one or more than one oils and light mist it on your bed. Let it dry in natural air and the dust mites will be out of your life.

- Use a good quality HEPA vacuum cleaner to clear all dust mites around you.

Recipe 18: Peppermint Essential Oil for Mice

Peppermint oil will be a great choice to get rid of mice in an area. You can use this oil in a diffuser in different areas of your house. Make sure to use pure oil and simply put a few drops oil on cotton balls. Keep these balls in different areas of your house. Peppermint oil may dispel quickly on a cotton ball so replace them twice a week.

Precautions for An Accident with Essential Oils

If an essential oil falls into your eyes accidentally, the immediately flush it with cold milk or vegetable oil to dilute the oil. If you still feel any stinging, you can consult a doctor immediately.

You can use cream or vegetable oil to remove the additional essential oils from your skin. Use soap and warm water to remove additional oil from the skin.

If you ingest any essential oil accidently, then you can call national poison control center for assistance.

Safety Tips for Massage Therapists

Extended exposure of essential oil can be the reason of nausea, headaches and irritation. If you want to avoid these feelings, then drink plenty of water and take frequent breaks.

It is not good to drive a vehicle immediately after a relaxing treatment and after the use of soporific oils like clary or sage.

If you are using essential oils for two weeks, then it is time to give a break for one week before continuing the use of oil. It will reduce the chances of any sensitive reaction.

If you are feeling soreness or cracks on the hands, then don't use sensitizing oils.

Essential Oils in the Pregnancy

There are lots of essential oils that can be safely inhaled and used on the surface of the skin in the pregnancy. It is important to be careful because the excessive quantity and misuses of essential oils can be the reason of potential damage. In the small quality, the oil will not harm you.

It is good to consult a licensed health practitioner before the use of essential oils. There are a few essential oils, such as Juniperus sabina (Savin) and Juniperus PFI Tze Riana (Spanish Sage) that should be avoided in the pregnancy. These can harm the unborn in the womb of a mother. Some other oils like Brazilian sassafras, Ocotea camphor, Chinese sassafras, Cinnamomum camphora should also be avoided during pregnancy.

Chapter 5 – Natural and Non-Toxic Repellent for Kids and Pets

There are a few sprays that you can use for pets and kids to keep insects away without harming their sensitive skin:

Recipe 19: Palo Santo Essential Oil

The palo santo essential oil is used to manage anger because its scent can keep insects away. Its anti-inflammatory properties can help you to avoid cancer as well. The regular use of this oil will help you to manage anger and stress.

Directions:

- 5 drops Cedarwood Atlas

- 4 drops Palo Santo

- 1 drop Patchouli

- 5 drops of Bergamot

Make a blend of these essential oils and apply it on the palms of your hands before going to head. Rub your hands and take a deep breath. You can massage your lower back and sole of the feet with the tips of your finger. You will notice a great difference in your condition after taking a massage with this blend.

Recipe 20: Peppermint Essential Oils

If you want to enhance your energy and confidence, then the peppermint essential oil will be an excellent drug for you. There is no need to drink caffeine because the essential oil can increase your energy levels. The peppermint oil trickles the freshness and improves your mental health. It can keep you alert and enables you to tackle each task in a better way.

Directions:

Peppermint essential oil can uplift your mood and confidence. You can include a few drops of peppermint oil in your bath water to keep your mind fresh. It will reduce tension, anxiety and enhance the feelings of calmness. In the absence of tension and anxiety, you can perform in a better way.

Recipe 21: Sandalwood Essential Oil

If you have dry or irritated skin, then you may feel low in the public places because a smooth and beautiful skin can boost your confidence. With dull and dry skin, you will only think about the negative views of people about you. If you want a glowing and healthy skin, then you should add a few drops of sandalwood essential oil in your body lotion. It will make your skin healthy and increase its glow. When you feel good in your own skin, your self-confidence will be at a higher level.

Recipe 22: Bergamot Essential Oil

The bergamot essential oil is an excellent addition to your daily routine because it can improve the health of your skin. It is often used in the production of perfumes and has amazing healing powers.

This oil is equally good for your brain because it can cure your stress, tension, and anger in a better way. If you want to increase your self-confidence, you should reduce your stress, anxiety, and tension. The Bergamot essential oil will play an important role in this.

Recipe 23: Rosemary Essential Oil

If you want to boost your confidence, then you should focus on your personal improvement. The rosemary essential oil will increase the shine and smooth texture of your hair. Just add five drops of rosemary oil in the bottle of shampoo. It will make your hair silky and keep your scalp free from dandruff. If you are suffering from migraines, then instead of using tablets, try this oil. Use a drop of this oil and massage on your wrists. Take q few deep breaths and feel the calm sensation.

Recipe 24: Tea Tree Essential Oil

If you are feeling any problem just because of virus and bacteria around you, then you should use tea tree oil. The oil will serve as a body bouncer and improve the immune system of your body in a natural way. It will save your money because after using this, there is no need to use expensive treatments. You can pamper your skin with the help of this oil because it may reduce the acne from your skin.

Tea tree oil will be an ultimate solution of your all problems. Take a bath by adding a few drops of tea tree essential oils in water.

Recipe 25: Chamomile Essential Oil

It is quite surprising to know that the chamomile is an excellent mood booster. If you are feeling burdened and want to get rid of these feelings, then use this oil. It is good to get rid of insects. Just add a few drops of chamomile oil in the boiling water, and take a bath to see its magic.

Ylang-Ylang Essential Oil

If you have ylang-ylang essential oil, then you can turn your own bathroom into a spa by adding a few drops of this oil in water. This will help you to control your emotions, and you may feel relaxed. This essential oil is available in a small bottle, and you can use it in different ways.

If you don't want to take a bath, then you can add a few drops in a very small bottle and spray this water on your face. It will enhance the feelings of calmness and relaxation. This is an excellent mood booster and increases your self-confidence as well.

There are lots of powerful essential oils that can increase your self-confidence and enhance your mood. You can inhale these oils or take a bath by adding a few drops. If you want to enjoy enough benefits of essential oils, then find the right oil for you to restore your energy. It will increase your self-confidence by boosting your mood.

Tips to Use Essential Oils for Different Purposes

If you want to enjoy all benefits of essential oils, it is important to use them accurately. In order to treat depression and anxiety with essential oil, you can follow given below directions:

Diffuse

It is important to use essential oils in diffused form by adding a few drops of the diffuser. If you want a better solution, then diffuse the essential oil in the night and use it before going to bed to get rid of additional thoughts. You can also put a few drops of oil on your pillow to inhale essential oils.

Inhalation

You can inhale the essential oils for better results. You just need to add a few drops of essential oil into the palm of your hand. Rub your hands together to spread the oil. Almost 4 to 6 deep breaths are enough. It will reduce the feeling of stress, depression and anxiety.

If you want to take a bath, then add 2 to 4 drops of essential oils in the water. It will reduce the feelings of depression, stress and anxiety. You need to include these essential oils to keep your body free from any trouble.

Massage:

You can take a massage by diffusing the essential oil with a carrier like a jojoba oil, grapeseed oil, sweet almond and other similar oils. Take the mixture and rub onto your chest, behind the ears, neck, wrists and ceiling of the feet.

Enjoy a Relaxing Bath

If you want to treat stress, depression and anxiety, then you can add 5 to 10 drops of essential oil in the bathtub. It can help you a lot, but for sensitive skin, you have to use diluted essential oils. Add these oils before and after a bath for better results.

Enjoy the Powerful Fragrance of Essential Oils

- You can surround yourself with a few drops of oil in your bottle of lotion.
- Keep in your car and house by placing a cotton ball of an essential oil at your place.
- You can put a few drops of essential oil on your favorite clothes.

Amazing Blend for Calm Mind

- 4 parts ylang-ylang EO
- 4 parts clary sage EO

- 2 parts basil EO

- 3 parts geranium EO

- 1 part sandalwood EO

Combine all these essential oils in a small bottle made of glass. It is important to choose a dark bottle to avoid oxidation. Take 1 to 2 drops on your palm and inhale the vapors. This blend can be included in the massage oils and bath tub.

Note: You are advised to choose only quality oils that should be 100% organic. These oils are made through non-chemical processes like steam distillation. These are safe for external and internal use.

Conclusion

Chemical based insect repellents can be too strong with harmful substances. There is no need to use chemical bug repellents because you can make your own natural repellent get rid of bugs and insects.

The homemade spray is the best alternative of commercial repellents. You can make a blend of different types of oils, lotions, and other items. Homemade insect sprays are free from toxins and you can use them without any danger.

With the help of essential oils, you can make a spray with the pleasant smell to keep the insects at bay. These sprays will provide a pleasant smell to your home and always keep you calm. There are numerous herbs and essential oils that can be used to get the advantage of its amazing smell.

There are numerous ways to get the advantage of plants around your house. It is essential to use these natural ingredients to design these sprays. This book is designed for your assistance with a lot of natural and non-toxic ant and mosquito repellents.

FREE Bonus Reminder

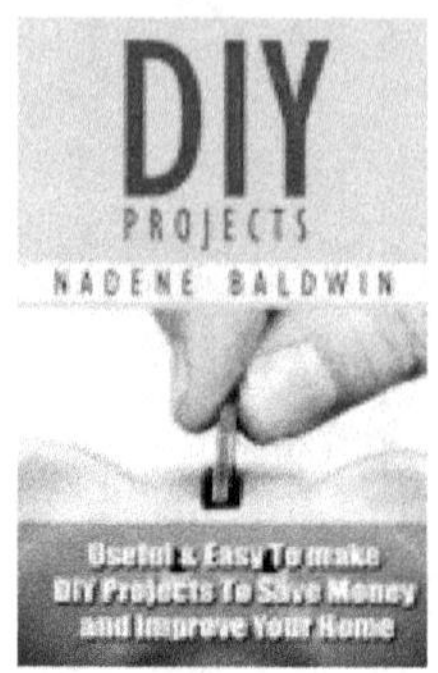

If you have not grabbed it yet, please go ahead and download your special bonus report *"DIY Projects. 13 Useful & Easy To Make DIY Projects To Save Money & Improve Your Home!"*

Simply Click the Button Below

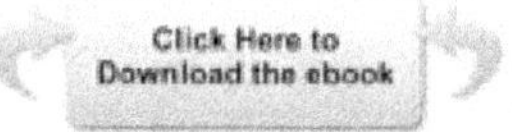

OR **Go to This Page**

http://diyhomecraft.com/free

BONUS #2: More Free & Discounted Books

Do you want to receive more Free & Discounted Books?

We have a mailing list where we send out our new Books when they go free or with a discount on Kindle. Click on the link below to sign up for Free & Discount Book Promotions.

=> Sign Up for Free & Discount Book Promotions <=

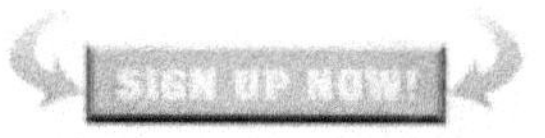

OR Go to this URL

http://zbit.ly/1WBb1Ek